The Sirtfood Diet Cookbook Recipes for Dinner

50 tasty and delicious recipes to end the day in the right way

Anne Patel

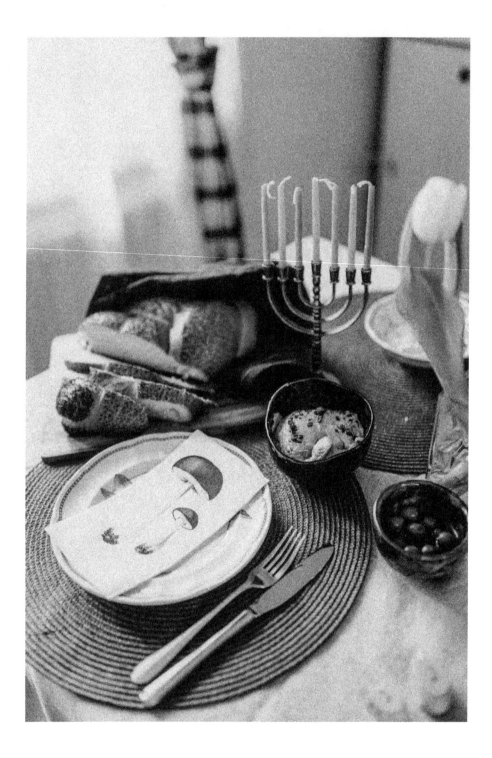

sources. Please consult a licensed professional before attempting any techniques outlined in this book.

By reading this document, the reader agrees that under no circumstances is the author responsible for any losses, direct or indirect, which are incurred as a result of the use of information contained within this document, including, but not limited to, — errors, omissions, or inaccuracies.

Table of Contents

Chapter 1: What is the Sirtfood diet

The Sirtfood Diet was created by Masters in Nutritional Medicine, Aiden Goggins and Glen Matten.

Their goal initially was to find a healthier way for people to eat, but people started losing weight quickly when they tested their program. With all the people in the world following diets hoping to lose pounds, they thought it would be selfish not to disclose their innovative health plan.

The plan they developed focuses on combining certain foods eaten in order to maximize the supply of nutrition to our body. There is an initial phase in which calories are limited to give the body a period to recover and eliminate accumulated waste. A maintenance phase follows this first phase to accustom the metabolism to the new foods you are ingesting. Throughout all stages, you will incorporate potent green juices and well-structured, well-planned meals.

The diet focuses on so-called 'sirtfoods,' plant-based foods that are known to stimulate a gene called sirtuin in the human body. Sirtuins belong to an entire protein family, called SIRT1 to

SIRT7, and each has specific health-related connections. These proteins help separate and safeguard our cells from inflammation and other damage resulting from everyday activities, helping to reduce our risk of developing major diseases, particularly those related to aging.

Studies have shown that people live longer and healthier lives when they eat diets rich in these foods that activate sirtuin, free from diabetes, heart disease, and even dementia. So this diet was designed to restore a healthy body situation, and one of the byproducts of a healthy body is also the loss of excess weight.

The diet Sirtfood is neither a miracle cure nor a week-long program designed to quickly lose weight before beach holidays. If you are only interested in losing a few pounds and then returning to your old habits, there are certainly plans and diets that are more suited to your needs.

The Sirtfood diet is a project born to help you for the rest of your life, using delicious foods, but that will also improve your health. If you switch from a standard American diet (SAD) to a sirtfood diet, you will lose all the weight your body does not need.

A healthy body does not store extra energy. It asks for what it needs and uses it effectively.

The diet isn't designed to encourage you to starve or deprive yourself. The fact is, foods that are deficient in nutrients are designer made to deprive you and, though the calories are there in plenty, your cells are still starved for the nutrition to help you thrive. The Sirtfood Diet is the opposite of deprivation and starvation. It is nourishment and balance.

Most people following the SAD may use 20 ingredients in a month, let alone enjoy the sheer volume of choice ingredients from the 120 options you will learn about here.

In recent decades, an alarming number of people have come to the conclusion that healthy food is boring, and plants or, more specifically, vegetables are terrible tasting. This is because the foods we've become dependent on – packed with sugar, salt, and unhealthy fats – have chemically altered our connection to food. Our brains are essentially lying to us, and our taste buds have been compromised.

This is one of the reasons the week-long reset is so important. After this first week, you will be able to taste food differently. The more you expose yourself to the recommended plant-based foods, the more pleasure you get out of them.

Sirtuins are critical for our health, regulating many essential biological functions, including our metabolism, which, I'm sure you know, is very closely connected to our weight. It's also a key figure in determining our body composition, such as how much muscle we build and how much fat we retain.

Sirtuin genes regulate all this and more. They're also integral in the process of aging and disease.

If we can turn these genes on, we'll be able to protect our cells and enjoy better health for longer life. Eating sirtfoods is the most effective way to accomplish this goal.

Sirtfoods are all plant-based, and they have many more benefits, in addition to being sirtuin activators.

Our bodies require energy to operate, and the majority of this fuel comes from three primary macronutrients: carbohydrates, fats, and proteins. These macros largely control our metabolic system and regulate how the calories we consume get processed by our bodies. This is why most diets focus exclusively on micronutrition and require you to calculate calories.

Our bodies need more than just energy to survive than thriving, however, which is why micronutrients are so important. They don't impact our weight as obviously as macros, but they are our health foundations.

Micronutrients, such as vitamins, minerals, fiber, antioxidants, and phytonutrients, are supposed to be consumed along with our calories. Unfortunately, in the Standard American Diet (SAD), they're in very limited supply.

When your diet is primarily made up of large quantities of red meat and processed meats, pre-packaged foods, vegetable oils, refined grains and a lot of sugar, you will have an almost total lack of micronutrition.

Plant foods offer the most micronutrients per calorie consumed. Every edible plant has a unique nutritional profile, protecting you from an innumerable variety of illnesses.

Sirtfoods, and other plant-based sources of nutrition, give your body what it needs to stay young and disease-free, and, as a bonus, this will help you remain at an ideal weight.

The original Sirtfood Diet encourages you to commit to a one week reset phase and then a 2-week maintenance phase where you rely heavily on the Sirtfood green juice for a significant dose of nutrition along with meals rich in sirtfoods. Once the phases are complete, to retain your health for the rest of your life, you will need to continue incorporating these sirtfoods into your daily meals.

The Sirtfood Diet is not a miracle cure, but if you stick to these recipes, you'll not just impress your taste buds, but you'll also enhance nearly every aspect of your health. To get safe, you don't have to count calories or starve yourself, the youthful body you've always wanted.

Sirtfood Diet Phases

Every newbie needs to understand that the sirtfood diet does not start with a single list of ingredients in your hands. Its implementation and adaptation are more than mere selective grocery shopping. Every diet can only work effectively when we allow our body to embrace the sudden shift and change in food intake. Similarly, the sirtfood diet also comes with two phases of adaptation. If a dieter successfully goes through these phases, he can continue with the sirtfood diet easily. There are mainly two phases of this diet, which are then succeeded by a third phase in which you can decide how you want to continue the diet.

Phase One

The first seven days of this diet plan are characterized as Phase One. In this phase, a dieter must focus on calorie restriction and the intake of green juices. These seven days are crucial to initiate your weight loss and usually help to lose up to seven pounds if the diet is followed properly. If you find yourself achieving this target, that means that you are on the right track.

In the first three days of the first phase, a dieter must restrict this caloric intake to 1,000 calories only. While doing so, the dieter must also have green juice throughout the day, probably three times a day. Try to drink green juice per meal. The recipes given in the book are perfect for selecting from.

Many meal options can keep your caloric intake in checks, such as buckwheat noodles, seared tofu, some shrimp stir fry, or sirtfood omelet.

Once the first three days of this diet has passed, you can increase your caloric intake to 1,500 calories per day. In these next four days, you can reduce the green juices to two times per side. And pair the juices with more Sirtuin-rich food in every meal.

Phase Two

After the first week of the sirtfood diet, then starts phase two. This phase is more about the maintenance of the diet, as the first week enables the body to embrace the change and start working according to the new diet. This phase enables the body to continue working towards the weight loss objective slowly and steadily. Therefore, the duration of this phase is almost two weeks.

So how is this phase different from phase one? In this phase, there is no restriction on the caloric intake, as long as the food is rich in sirtuins and you are taking it three times a day, it is good to go. Instead of having the green juice two or three times a day, the dieter can have juice one time a day, and that will be enough to achieve steady weight loss. You can have the juice after any meal, in the morning or in the evening.

After the Diet Phase

With the end of phase two comes the time, which is most crucial, and that is the after-diet phase. If your weight loss target has not been reached by the end of step two, then you can restart the phases all over again. Or even when you have achieved the goals but still want to lose more weight, then you can again give it a try.

Instead of following phases one and two over and over again, you can also continue having good quality sirtfood meals in this after-diet phase. Simply continue the eating practices of phase two, have a diet rich in sirtuin and do have green juices whenever possible. The diet is mainly divided into two phases: the first lasts one week, and the other lasts 14 days.

The best 20 sirt foods

All these foods include high quantities of plant compounds called polyphenols, which can be thought to modify the sirtuin enzymes, therefore, excite their super-healthy added benefits.

Top 20 sirtfoods

1. Arugula (Rocket)
2. Buckwheat
3. Capers
4. Celery
5. Chilis
6. Cocoa
7. Coffee
8. Extra Virgin Olive Oil
9. Garlic
10. Green Tea (especially Matcha)
11. Kale
12. Medjool Dates
13. Parsley
14. Red Endive
15. Red Onions
16. Red Wine
17. Soy
18. Strawberries

19. Turmeric

20. Walnuts

What Is So Great About Sirtuins?

There are seven types of Sirtuins named from **SIRT1** to **SIRT7**. Although our understanding of the exact functions of all the Sirtuins is minimal, studies show that activating them can have the following benefits:

Switching on fat burning and protection from weight gain: Sirtuins do this by increasing the mitochondrion's functionality (which is involved in the production of energy) and sparking a change in your metabolism to break down more fat cells.

Improving Memory by protecting neurons from damage. Sirtuins also boost learning skills and memory through the enhancement of synaptic plasticity. Synaptic plasticity refers to synapses' capacity to weaken or strengthen with time due to decreased or increased activity. This is important because memories are represented by different interconnected networks of synapses in the brain, and synaptic plasticity is an important neurochemical foundation of memory and learning.

Slowing down the Ageing Process: Sirtuins act as cell guarding enzymes. Thus, they protect the cells and slow down their aging process.

Repairing cells: The Sirtuins repair cells damaged by re-activating cell functionality.

Protection against diabetes: this happens through prevention against insulin resistance. Sirtuins do this by controlling blood sugar levels because this diet calls for moderate consumption of carbohydrates. These foods cause increases in blood sugar levels; hence the need to release insulin, and as the blood sugar levels increase greatly, there is a need to produce more insulin. Over time, cells become resistant to insulin, hence producing more insulin and leading to insulin resistance.

Fighting Cancers: The chemicals working as sirtuin activators affect the function of sirtuin in different cells, i.e. by switching it on when in normal cells and shutting it down in cancerous cells. This encourages the death of cancerous cells.

Fighting inflammation: Sirtuins have a powerful antioxidant effect that has the power to reduce oxidative stress. This has positive effects on heart health and cardiovascular protection.

Chapter 2: How do the Sirtfood Diet Works?

The basis of the sirtuin diet can be explained in simple terms or in complex ways. However, it's important to understand how and why it works so that you can appreciate the value of what you are doing. It is important to also know why these sirtuin rich foods help to help you maintain fidelity to your diet plan. Otherwise, you may throw something in your meal with less nutrition that would defeat the purpose of planning for one rich in sirtuins. Most importantly, this is not a dietary fad, and as you will see, there is much wisdom contained in how humans have used natural foods, even for medicinal purposes, over thousands of years.

To understand how the Sirtfood diet works and why these particular foods are necessary, we're going to look at their role in the human body.

Sirtuin activity was first researched in yeast, where a mutation caused an extension in the yeast's lifespan. Sirtuins were also shown to slow aging in laboratory mice, fruit flies, and nematodes. As research on Sirtuins proved to transfer to mammals, they were examined for their use in diet and slowing the aging process. The sirtuins in humans are different in typing, but they essentially work in the same ways and reasons.

The Sirtuin family is made up of seven "members." It is believed that sirtuins play a big role in regulating certain functions of cells, including proliferation, reproduction and growth of cells), apoptosis death of cells). They promote survival and resist stress to increase longevity.

They are also seen to block neurodegeneration loss or function of the nerve cells in the brain). They conduct their housekeeping functions by cleaning out toxic proteins and supporting the brain's ability to change and adapt to different conditions or to recuperate i.e., brain plasticity). They also help minimize chronic inflammation as part of this and decrease anything called oxidative stress. Oxidative stress is when there are so many free radicals present in the body that are cell-damaging, and by fighting them with antioxidants, the body can not keep up. These factors are related to age-related illness and weight as well, which again brings us back to a discussion of how they actually work.

You will see labels in Sirtuins that start with "SIR," which represents "Silence Information Regulator" genes. They do exactly that, silence or regulate, as part of their functions. Humans work with the seven sirtuins: SIRT1, SIRT2, SIRT3,

SIRT4, SIRT 5, SIRT6 and SIRT7. Each of these types is responsible for different areas of protecting cells. They work by either stimulating or turning on certain gene expressions or by reducing and turning off other gene expressions. This essentially means that they can influence genes to do more or less of something, most of which they are already programmed to do.

Through enzyme reactions, each of the SIRT types affects different areas of cells responsible for the metabolic processes that help maintain life. This is also related to what organs and functions they will affect.

For example, the SIRT6 causes and expression of genes in humans that affect skeletal muscle, fat tissue, brain, and heart. SIRT 3 would cause an expression of genes that affect the kidneys, liver, brain and heart.

If we tie these concepts together, you can see that the Sirtuin proteins can change the expression of genes, and in the case of the Sirtfood diet, we care about how sirtuins can turn off those genes that are responsible for speeding up aging and for weight management.

The other aspect to this conversation of sirtuins is the function and the power of calorie restriction on the human body. Calorie restriction is simply eating fewer calories. This, coupled with exercise and reducing stress, is usually a combination for weight loss. Calorie restriction has also proven across much research in animals and humans to increase one's lifespan.

We can look further at the role of sirtuins with calorie restriction and using the SIRT3 protein, which has a role in metabolism and aging. Amongst all of the effects of the protein on gene expression, such as preventing cells from dying, reducing tumors from growing, etc.), we want to understand the effects of SIRT3 on weight for this book's purpose.

As we stated earlier, the SIRT3 has high expression in those metabolically active tissues, and its ability to express itself increases with caloric restriction, fasting, and exercise. On the contrary, it will express itself less when the body has high fat, high calorie-riddled diet.

The last few highlights of sirtuins are their role in regulating telomeres and reducing inflammation, which also helps with staving off disease and aging.
Telomeres are sequences of proteins at the ends of chromosomes. When cells divide, these get shorter. As we age, they get shorter, and other stressors to the body also will contribute to this. Maintaining these longer telomeres is the key to slower aging. In addition, proper diet, along with exercise and other variables, can lengthen telomeres. SIRT6 is one of the

sirtuins that, if activated, can help with DNA damage, inflammation and oxidative stress. SIRT1 also helps with inflammatory response cycles that are related to many age-related diseases.

Calories restriction can extend life to some degree. Since this and fasting are a stressor, these factors will stimulate the SIRT3 proteins to kick in and protect the body from the stressors and excess free radicals. Again, the telomere length is affected as well.

Having laid this all out before you, you should appreciate how and why these miraculous compounds work in your favor, keep you youthful, healthy, and lean If they are working hard for you, don't you feel that you should do something too?

50 Essential Dinner Recipes

1. Carrot, Buckwheat, Tomato & Arugula Salad in a Jar

Preparation time: 5 Minutes

Cooking Time: 30 Minutes

Servings 2

Ingredients

1/2 cup sunflower seeds

1/2 cup carrots

1/2 cup of shredded cabbage

1/2 cup of tomatoes

1 cup cooked buckwheat mixed with 1 tbsp. chia seeds

1 cup arugula

Dressing:

1 tbsp. olive oil

1 tbsp. fresh lemon juice and pinch of sea salt

Directions:

1. Put ingredients in this order: dressing, sunflower seeds, carrots, cabbage, tomatoes, buckwheat and arugula.

2. Honey Mustard Dressing

Preparation time: 10 minutes

Cooking time: 0 minutes

Servings: 2

Ingredients:

4 tablespoon Olive oil

11/2 teaspoon Honey

11/2 teaspoon Mustard

1 teaspoon Lemon juice

1 pinch Salt

Directions:

Mix olive oil, honey, mustard and lemon juice into an even dressing with a whisk.

Season with salt.

3. Warm tomato salad

Preparation time: 5 Minutes

Cooking Time: 10 Minutes

Servings: 4-5

Ingredients:

4 tomatoes, sliced

1 cup cherry tomatoes, halved

½ small red onion, very finely cut

2 garlic cloves, crushed

1 tbsp dried mint

2 tbsp extra virgin olive oil

1 tbsp balsamic vinegar

Directions:

Gently heat oil in a nonstick frying pan over low heat. Cook garlic and tomatoes, stirring occasionally, for 4-5 Minutes or until tomatoes are warm but firm. Remove from heat and place in a plate.

Add in red onion, vinegar and dried mint. To taste and serve, season with salt and pepper.

4. Shredded kale and brussels sprout salad

Preparation time: 10 Minutes

Cooking Time: 20 Minutes

Servings: 4-6

Ingredients:

18-29 brussels sprouts, shredded

1 cup finely shredded kale

1/2 cup grated parmesan or pecorino cheese 1 cup walnuts, halved, toasted

1/2 cup dried cranberries

For the dressing:

6 tbsp extra virgin olive oil

2 tbsp apple cinder vinegar

1 tbsp dijon mustard

Salt and pepper, to taste

Directions:

Shred the brussels sprouts and kale in a food processor or mandolin. Toss them in a bowl, top with toasted walnuts, cranberries and grated cheese.

Whisk in the olive oil in a smaller cup, apple cider vinegar and mustard until smooth. Pour over the salad with the sauce, stir and eat.

5. Quinoa and zucchini ribbon salad

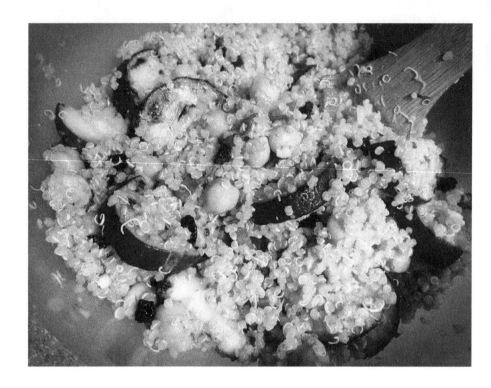

Preparation time: 10 Minutes

Cooking Time: 40 Minutes

Servings: 4

Ingredients:

1 cup quinoa

2 cups water

1 zucchini, sliced lengthways into thin ribbons (a mandoline is ideal)

3-4 green onions, chopped

1 cup cherry tomatoes, halved

4 oz feta, crumbled or cut in small cubes

2 tbsp extra virgin olive oil

3 tbsp lemon juice

Salt, to taste

Directions:

Heat oil over medium to high heat in a large saucepan. Add zucchini and and cook, stirring, until zucchini is crisp-tender, about 4 minutes. Set aside in a plate.

Wash the quinoa for 1-2 minutes in a fine mesh strainer under running water, then set aside to drain. Bring water to the boil in a medium saucepan over high heat. Attach the quinoa and put it back to the boil. Cover and cook gently, reducing the heat to a simmer, for 15 minutes. Put aside for 5-6 minutes, sealed.

Toss quinoa with zucchini, green onions, tomatoes, lemon juice and olive oil.

Serve warm or at room temperature, with feta cheese topping.

6. Kale white bean pork soup

Preparation time: 5 Minutes

Cooking Time: 45 Minutes

Servings 4-6

Ingredients - allergies: sf, gf, df, ef, nf

3 tbsp. Extra-virgin olive oil

3 tbsp. Chili powder

1 tbsp. Jalapeno hot sauce

2 pounds bone-in pork chops

Salt

4 stalks celery, chopped

1 large white onion, chopped

3 cloves garlic, chopped

2 cups chicken broth

2 cups diced tomatoes

2 cups cooked white beans

6 cups packed kale

Directions

Preheat the broiler. Whisk hot sauce, 1 tbsp. Olive oil in a bowl and chili powder. Season the pork chops with 1/2 tsp. Salt. Rub chops with the spice mixture on both sides and place them on a rack set over a baking sheet. Set aside.

Heat 1 tbsp. Olive oil in a pot over medium heat. Add the celery, garlic, onion and the remaining 2 tbsp. Chili powder. Cook until onions are translucent, stirring (approx. 8 minutes).

Add tomatoes and the chicken broth to the pot. Cook and stir occasionally until reduced by about one-third (approx.7 minutes). Add the kale and the beans. Decrease the heat to medium, cover and cook until the kale is soft (approx. 7 minutes). If the mixture looks dry, add up to half a cup of water and season with salt.

In the meantime, broil the pork until browned (approx. 4 to 6 minutes). Flip and broil until cooked through. Serve with the kale and beans.

7. Turkey satay skewers

Ingredients

250g (9oz) turkey breast, cubed 25g (1oz) smooth peanut butter
1 clove of garlic, crushed
½ small bird's eye chilli (or more if you like it hotter), finely
chopped ½ teaspoon ground turmeric
200mls (7fl oz) coconut milk 2 teaspoons soy sauce

Servings 2
431 calories per serving

Directions

Combine the coconut milk, peanut butter, turmeric, soy sauce, garlic and chilli. Add the turkey pieces to the bowl and stir them until they are completely coated. Push the turkey onto metal skewers. Place the satay skewers on a barbeque or under a hot grill (broiler) and Cook on each side for 4-5 minutes, until fully cooked.

8. Salmon & capers

Ingredients

75g (3oz) greek yogurt

4 salmon fillets, skin removed 4 teaspoons dijon mustard

1 tablespoon capers, chopped 2 teaspoons fresh parsley

Zest of 1 lemon

Servings 4

321 calories per serving

Directions

Mix the yogurt, mustard, lemon zest, parsley and capers together in a dish. Thoroughly coat the salmon in the mixture. Place the salmon under a hot grill (broiler) and cook for 3-4 minutes on each side, or until the fish is cooked. Serve with mashed potatoes and vegetables or a large green leafy salad.

9. Buckwheat and nut loaf

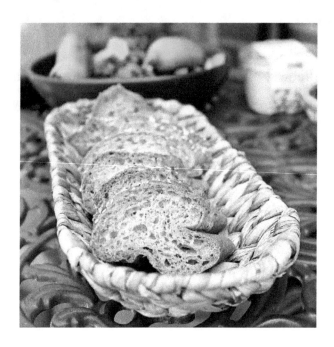

Preparation Time: 15 minutes

Cooking Time: 30 minutes

Servings: 4

Ingredients:

225g/8oz buckwheat

2 tbsp. olive oil

225g/8oz mushrooms

2-3 carrots, finely diced

2-3 tbsp. fresh herbs, finely chopped e.g., oregano, marjoram, thyme and parsley

225g/8oz nuts e.g., hazelnuts, almonds, walnuts

2 eggs, beaten (or 2 tbsp. tahini for vegan version)

Salt and pepper

Directions:

1. First of all, put the buckwheat in a pan with 350ml/1.5 cups of water and a pinch of salt. Boil it.

2. Cover and boil with the lid on for about 10-15 minutes, until all the water has been absorbed.

3. Meanwhile, in the olive oil, sauté the mushrooms and carrots until tender.

4. Blitz the nuts until well chopped in the food processor.

5. Stir in the eggs and mix the carrots, cooked buckwheat, herbs and chopped nuts. Combine this with some water while using tahini instead of eggs to create a dense pouring consistency before stirring it into the buckwheat.

6. Season it with pepper and salt.

7. Move to a lined or oiled loaf tin and cook for 30 minutes in the oven on gas mark 5/190C until set and just browned on top.

Nutrition: Calories 163 Carbs 23g Protein 6g Fiber 4g

10. Vegetable broth

Preparation time: 5 Minutes

Cooking Time: 40 Minutes

Servings: 6 cups

Ingredients

1 tbsp. Olive oil

1 large red onion

2 stalks celery, including some leaves

2 large carrots

1 bunch green onions, chopped

8 cloves garlic, minced

8 sprigs fresh parsley

6 sprigs fresh thyme

2 bay leaves

1 tsp. Salt

2 quarts water

Directions - allergies: sf, gf, df, ef, v, nf

Chop veggies into small chunks. Add the onion, scallions, celery, carrots, garlic, parsley, thyme, and bay leaves and heat the oil in a soup pot. For 5 to 7 minutes, cook over high heat, stirring occasionally.

Bring it to a boil, then add salt to it. Lower heat and boil 30 minutes, uncovered. Uh, strain. Other ingredients to consider: stalk of broccoli, root of celery

11. Chicken broth

Preparation time: 5 Minutes

Cooking Time: 50 Minutes

Servings 3

Ingredients

4 lbs. Fresh chicken (wings, necks, backs, legs, bones)

2 peeled onions or 1 cup chopped leeks

2 celery stalks

1 carrot

8 black peppercorns

2 sprigs fresh thyme

2 sprigs fresh parsley

1 tsp. Salt

Directions - allergies: sf, gf, df, ef, nf

Put cold water in a stock pot and add chicken. Bring just to a boil. Skim any foam from the surface. Add other ingredients, return just to a boil, and reduce heat to a slow simmer. Simmer for 2 hours. Let cool and strain until room temperature is warm. Keep the broth cool and use or freeze it within a few days. Defrost and boil prior to use.

12. Artichoke, Chicken and Capers

Preparation time: 10 minutes

Cooking time: 55 minutes

Servings: 2

Ingredients

6 boneless, skinless chicken breasts

2 cups mushrooms, sliced

1 (14 ½ ounce) can diced tomatoes

1 (8 or 9 ounce) package frozen artichokes

1 cup chicken broth

¼ cup dry white wine

1 medium yellow onion, diced

½ cup Kalamata olives, sliced ¼ cup capers, drained

3 tablespoons chia seeds

3 teaspoons curry powder

1 teaspoon turmeric

3/4 teaspoon dried lovage Salt and pepper to taste

3 cups hot cooked buckwheat

Directions
Rinse chicken & set aside.

In a large bowl, combine mushrooms, tomatoes – with juice, frozen artichoke hearts, chicken broth, white wine, onion, olives and capers.

Stir in chia seeds, curry powder, turmeric, lovage, salt and pepper.
Pour half the mixture into your crockpot, add the chicken, and pour the remainder of the sauce overtop.

Cover and bake for 7 to 8 hours on low or 3 1/2 to 4 hours on high.

Serve with hot cooked buckwheat.

13. Quinoa and avocado salad

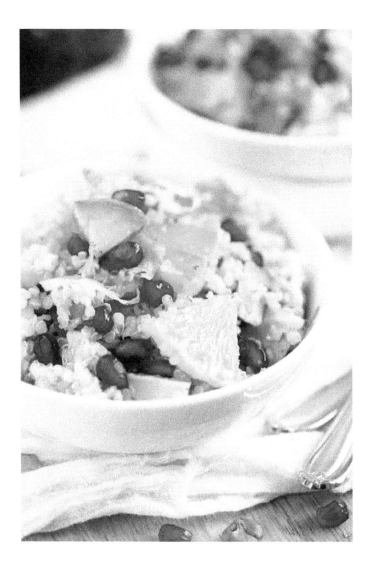

Preparation time: 10 Minutes

Cooking Time: 20 Minutes

Servings: 4

Ingredients:

1 cup quinoa

2 cups water

1 large avocado, pitted and sliced

¼ radicchio, finely sliced

1 small pink grapefruit, peeled and finely cut

1 handful arugula

1 cup baby spinach leaves

2 tbsp extra virgin olive oil

2 tbsp lemon juice

Salt and black pepper, to taste

Directions:

Wash quinoa in a fine sieve under running water for 2-3 minutes, or until water runs clear. Set aside to drain, then boil it in two cups of water for 15 minutes.

Fluff with a fork and put to cool aside. Stir avocado, radicchio, arugula and baby spinach into cooled quinoa.

Add grapefruit, lemon juice, and olive oil, season with salt and black pepper and stir to combine well.

14. Quinoa and carrot salad

Preparation time: 10 Minutes

Cooking Time: 0 Minutes

Servings: 4

Ingredients:

1 cup quinoa

2 cups water

4 carrots, shredded

1 apple, peeled and shredded

1 garlic clove, chopped

3 tbsp lemon juice

2 tbsp extra virgin olive oil

Salt, to taste

Directions:

In a sieve under running water, rinse the quinoa very well and set aside to drain. Boil two cups of water add in quinoa and simmer for 15 minutes. Fluff with a fork and set aside to cool.

In a deep salad bowl, combine the shredded carrots, apple and lemon juice, garlic and salt. Add in the cooled quinoa, toss to combine and serve.

15. Quinoa, kale and roasted pumpkin

Preparation time: 10 Minutes

Cooking Time: 20 Minutes

Servings: 4-5

Ingredients:

1 cup quinoa

2 cups water

1.5 lb pumpkin, peeled and seeded, cut into cubes

2 cups fresh kale, chopped

5 oz crumbled feta cheese

1 large onion, finely chopped

4-5 tbsp extra virgin olive oil

1 tsp finely grated ginger

½ tsp cumin

½ tsp salt

Directions:

Preheat oven to 350 f. Line a baking tray and arrange the pumpkin cubes on on it. Drizzle with 2-3 Tablespoons of olive oil and salt. Place in the oven and cook for 20-25 minutes, stirring every 10 minutes. Toss to cover.

Heat the remaining olive oil over a medium-high heat in a large saucepan. Sauté the onion gently for 2-3 minutes or until tender. Connect the spices and cook for 1 minute more, stirring.

Wash quinoa under running water until the water runs clear. Boil two cups of water and add the quinoa to the boil. Reduce heat to low, cover, and simmer for 15 minutes. Incorporate kale and cook until it wilts. Gently combine quinoa and kale mixture with the roasted pumpkin and sautéed onion.

16. Lamb, Butternut Squash and Date Tagine

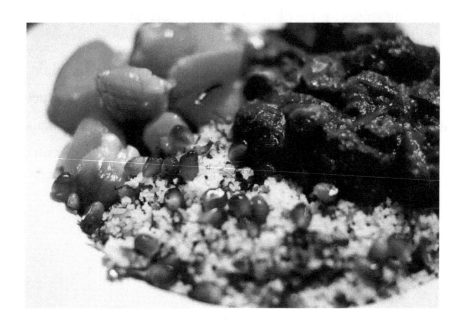

Preparation time: 10 minutes

Cooking time: 25 minutes

Servings: 2

Ingredients:

Two tablespoons olive oil

One red onion, cut

2cm ginger, ground

Three garlic cloves, ground or squashed

One teaspoon stew pieces (or to taste)

Two teaspoons cumin seeds

One cinnamon stick

Two teaspoons ground turmeric

800g sheep neck filet, cut into 2cm pieces

½ teaspoon salt

100g Medjool dates, hollowed and hacked

400g tin hacked tomatoes, in addition to a large portion of a container of water

500g butternut squash, chopped into 1cm 3D shapes

400g tin chickpeas, depleted

Two tablespoons new coriander (in addition to extra for decorate)

Buckwheat, couscous, flatbreads or rice to serve

Directions:

Preheat your stove to 140C.

Drizzle around two tablespoons of olive oil into an enormous ovenproof pot or cast iron meal dish. Include the cut onion and cook on a delicate warmth, with the cover on, for around 5 minutes, until the onions are mellowed however not dark-coloured.

Add the ground garlic and ginger, bean stew, cumin, cinnamon and turmeric. Mix well and cook for one increasingly minute with the cover off. Include a sprinkle of water if it gets excessively dry.

Next include the sheep pieces. Mix well to cover the onions and flavours with the beef and afterwards include the salt, hacked dates and tomatoes, in addition to about a large portion of a jar of water (100-200ml).

Bring the tagine to the bubble and afterwards put the cover on and put in your preheated stove for 1 hour and 15 minutes.

Thirty minutes before the finish of the cooking time, include the cleaved butternut squash and depleted chickpeas. Mix everything, set the cover back on and come back to the stove for the last 30 minutes of cooking.

When the tagine is prepared, expel from the stove and mix through the cleaved coriander. Present with buckwheat, couscous, flatbreads or basmati rice.

17. Prawn Arrabbiata

Preparation time: 10 minutes
Cooking time: 55 minutes
Servings: 2

Ingredients:

125-150 g Raw or cooked prawns (Ideally ruler prawns)
65 g Buckwheat pasta
1 tbsp Extra virgin olive oil

For arrabbiata sauce
40 g Red onion, finely slashed
1 Garlic clove, finely slashed
30 g Celery, finely slashed
1 Bird's eye bean stew, finely hacked
1 tsp Dried blended herbs
1 tsp Extra virgin olive oil
2 tbsp White wine (discretionary)
400 g Tinned slashed tomatoes
1 tbsp Chopped parsley

Directions:

Fry the onion, garlic, celery and bean stew and dried herbs in the oil over a medium-low warmth for 1–2 minutes. Turn the heat up to medium, include the wine and cook for one moment.

Include the tomatoes and leave the sauce to stew over a medium-low warmth for 20–30 minutes, until it has a pleasant creamy consistency. Only include a little water on the off chance that you thought the sauce is getting too thick.

While the sauce is cooking, carry a container of water to the bubble and cook the pasta as per the bundle guidelines. At the point when prepared just as you would prefer, channel, hurl with the olive oil and keep in the container until required.

Mix them into the sauce on the off that you are using crude prawns and bake for another 3-4 minutes until it has turned pink and dark,including the parsley and serve. If you are utilizing cooked prawns, include them with the parsley, carry the sauce to the bubble and help.

Add pasta to the sauce, blend altogether yet tenderly and serve.

18. Turmeric Baked Salmon

Preparation time: 10 minutes

Cooking time: 50 minutes

Servings: 2

Ingredients:

125-150 g Skinned Salmon

1 tsp Extra virgin olive oil

1 tsp ground turmeric

1/4 Juice of a lemon

For the fiery celery

1 tsp Extra virgin olive oil

40 g Red onion, finely slashed

60 g Tinned green lentils

1 Garlic clove, finely slashed

1 cm fresh ginger, finely slashed

1 Bier's eye bean stew, finely slashed

150 g Celery, cut into 2cm lengths

1 tsp Mild curry powder

130 g Tomato, cut into eight wedges

100 ml Chicken or vegetable stock

1 tbsp Chopped parsley

Directions:

Heat the grill to 200C/gas mark 6.

Start with the fiery celery. Warmth a skillet over medium-low heat, include the olive oil, at that point the onion, garlic, ginger, bean stew and celery. Fry tenderly for 2–3 minutes or until mollified however not hued, at that point include the curry powder and cook for a further moment.

Add the red tomato then the stock and lentils and stew delicately for 10 minutes. You might need to increment or decrease the cooking time contingent upon how crunchy you like your celery.

Meanwhile, blend the turmeric, oil and lemon squeeze and rub over the salmon.

Place on a heating plate and cook for 8–10 minutes.

To complete, mix the parsley through the celery and present with the salmon.

19. Buckwheat with Mushrooms and Green Onions

Preparation time: 10 minutes

Cooking time: 40 minutes

Servings: 2

Ingredients

1 cup buckwheat groats

2 cups vegetable or chicken broth

3 green onions, thinly sliced

1 cup mushrooms, sliced

Salt and pepper to taste

2 teaspoons butter

Directions

Combine all ingredients in your crockpot. Cover and cook on low for 4 to 4 1/2 hours.

20. Pasta with Cheesy Meat Sauce

Preparation Time: 10 minutes
Cooking Time: 30 minutes
Servings: 6

Ingredients:

½ box large-shaped pasta

1-pound ground beef*

½ cup onions, diced

1 tablespoon onion flakes

1½ cups beef stock, reduced or no sodium

1 tablespoon Better Than Bouillon® beef, no salt added

1 tablespoon tomato sauce, no salt added

¾ cup Monterey or pepper jack cheese, shredded

8 ounces cream cheese, softened

½ teaspoon Italian seasoning

½ teaspoon ground black pepper

2 tablespoons French's® Worcestershire sauce, reduced sodium

Directions:

1. Cook pasta noodles as per the directions on the box.

2. Cook the ground beef, onions and onion flakes in a large skillet until the meat is browned.

3. Add stock, bouillon and tomato sauce and drain.

4. Bring to a boil, sometimes stirring. Stir in the pasta that has been cooked, turn off the heat and add the cream cheese, shredded cheese and flavoured cheese (Italian seasoning, black pepper and Worcestershire sauce). Stir in the pasta mixture until all the cheese is melted.

TIP: You can substitute beef for ground turkey.

Nutrition: Calories: 502 kcal Total Fat: 30 g Saturated Fat: 14 g Cholesterol: 99 mg Sodium: 401 mg Total Carbs: 35 g Fiber: 1.7 g Sugar: 0 g Protein: 23 g

21. Kale, Apple, & Cranberry Salad

Preparation time: **15 minutes**

Cooking time: **5 minutes**

Servings: 4

Ingredients

6 cups fresh baby kale

3 large apples, cored and sliced

¼ cup unsweetened dried cranberries

¼ cup almonds, sliced

tablespoons extra-virgin olive oil

1 tablespoon raw honey

Salt and ground black pepper, to taste

Directions

1. Place all the ingredients in a salad bowl and toss to coat them well.

2. Serve immediately.

22. Arugula, Strawberry, & Orange Salad

Preparation time: **15 minutes**
Servings: 4

Ingredients

Salad
6 cups fresh baby arugula
1½ cups fresh strawberries, hulled and sliced 2 oranges, peeled and segmented

Dressing
2 tablespoons fresh lemon juice
1 tablespoon raw honey
2 teaspoons extra-virgin olive oil
1 teaspoon Dijon mustard
Salt and ground black pepper, to taste

Directions
For salad: in a salad bowl, place all ingredients and mix.

For dressing: place all ingredients in another bowl and beat until well combined.

Place dressing on top of salad and toss to coat well.

23. Minty Tomatoes and Corn

Preparation time: 10 minutes

Cooking time: 65 minutes

Servings: 2

Ingredients:

2 c. corn

1 tbsp. rosemary vinegar

2 tbsps. chopped mint

1 lb. sliced tomatoes

¼ tsp. black pepper

2 tbsps. olive oil

Directions:

In a salad bowl, combine the tomatoes with the corn and the other ingredients, toss and serve.

24. Beef & Kale Salad

Preparation time: **15 minutes**
Cooking time: **8 minutes**
Servings: 2

Ingredients
Steak
2 teaspoons olive oil
2 (4-ounce) strip steaks
Salt and ground black pepper, to taste

Salad
¼ cup carrot, peeled and shredded
¼ cup cucumber, peeled, seeded, and sliced
¼ cup radish, sliced
¼ cup cherry tomatoes, halved
3 cups fresh kale, tough ribs removed and chopped

Dressing
1 tablespoon extra-virgin olive oil
1 tablespoon fresh lemon juice
Salt and ground black pepper, to taste

Directions

1. For steak: in a large heavy-bottomed wok, heat the oil over high heat and cook the steaks with salt and black pepper for about 3–4 minutes per side.

2. Transfer the steaks onto a cutting board for about 5 minutes before slicing.

3. For salad: place all ingredients in a salad bowl and mix.

4. For dressing: place all ingredients in another bowl and beat until well combined.

5. Cut the steaks into desired sized slices against the grain.

6. Place the salad onto each serving plate.

7. Top each plate with steak slices.

8. Drizzle with dressing and serve.

25. Salmon Burgers

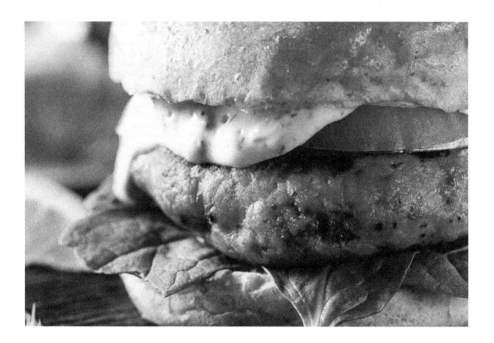

Preparation time: **20 minutes**

Cooking time: **15 minutes**

Servings: 5

Ingredients

Burgers

1 teaspoon olive oil

1 cup fresh kale, tough ribs removed and chopped 1/3 cup shallots, chopped finely

Salt and ground black pepper, to taste

16 ounces skinless salmon fillets

¾ cup cooked quinoa

2 tablespoons Dijon mustard

1 large egg, beaten

Salad

2½ tablespoons olive oil

2½ tablespoons red wine vinegar

Salt and ground black pepper, to taste

8 cups fresh baby arugula

2 cups cherry tomatoes, halved

Directions

1. For burgers: in a large non-stick wok, heat the oil over medium heat and sauté the kale, shallots, salt, and black pepper for about 4–5 minutes.

2. Remove from heat and transfer the kale mixture into a large bowl.

3. Set aside to cool slightly.

4. With a knife, chop 4 ounces of salmon and transfer into the bowl of kale mixture.

5. In a food processor, add the remaining salmon and pulse until finely chopped.

6. Transfer the finely chopped salmon into the bowl of kale mixture.

7. Then, add remaining ingredients and stir until fully combined.

8. Make 5 equal-sized patties from the mixture.

9. Heat a lightly greased large non-stick wok over medium heat and cook the patties for about 4–5 minutes per side.

10. For dressing: in a glass bowl, add the oil, vinegar, shallots, salt, and black pepper, and beat until well combined.

11. To coat well, add the arugula and tomatoes and toss.

12. Divide the salad onto on serving plates and top each with 1 patty.

13. Serve immediately.

26. Sirtfood bites

Ingredients:

4 oz walnuts

1 oz dark chocolate (85 per cent cocoa solids), broken into pieces; or cocoa nibs

9 oz Medjool dates, pitted 1 tbsp cocoa powder

1 tbsp ground turmeric

1 tbsp extra virgin vegetable oil the scraped seeds of 1 vanilla pod or 1 tsp vanilla 1–2 tbsp water

Directions:

Place the walnuts and chocolate during a kitchen appliance and process until you have a fine powder. Add all the opposite ingredients except the water and blend until the mixture forms a ball. Depending on the consistency of the mixture, you may or may not have to add water-you don't want it to be too wet. Shape the mixture into bite-sized balls using your hands and refrigerate for at least 1 hour in an airtight container before eating them. You'll roll some of the balls in some more cocoa or desiccated coconut to realize a different finish if you wish. They will keep for up to 1 week in your fridge.

27. Asian king prawn stir-fry with buckwheat noodles

Ingredients:

5 oz shelled raw king prawns, deveined

2 tsp tamari (you can use soy sauce if you're not avoiding gluten)

2 tsp extra virgin olive oil

2.5 oz soba (buckwheat noodles) 1 clove , finely chopped

1 bird's eye chilli, finely chopped 1 tsp finely chopped fresh ginger ¼ red onions, sliced

1.5 oz celery, trimmed and sliced 3 oz green beans, chopped

2 oz kale, roughly chopped

½ cup chicken broth

1 tbsp lovage or celery leaves

Directions:

Over a high heat, heat a frypan, then cook the prawns for 2-3 minutes in 1 teaspoon tamari and 1 teaspoon oil. Transfer the prawns to a plate. Wipe the pan out with kitchen paper, as you're getting to use it again. Cook the noodles in boiling water for 5–8 minutes or as directed on the packet. Drain and set aside.

Meanwhile, fry the garlic, chilli and ginger, red onion, celery, beans and kale within the remaining oil over an medium–high heat for 2–3 minutes. Add the stock and convey to the boil, then simmer for a minute or two, until the vegetables are cooked but still crunchy.

Add the prawns, noodles and lovage/celery leaves to the pan, bring back to the boil then remove from the heat and serve.

28. Strawberry buckwheat tabouleh

Ingredients:

2 oz buckwheat

1 tbsp ground turmeric

½ avocado

½ tomato

¼ red onion

1 oz Medjool dates, pitted

1 tbsp capers

1 oz parsley

3 oz strawberries, hulled

1 tbsp extra virgin olive oil

juce of ½ lemon

1 oz rocket

Directions:

Cook the buckwheat with the turmeric consistent with the packet instructions.

Drain and keep to one side to chill.

Finely chop the avocado, tomato, red onion, dates, capers and parsley and blend with the cool buckwheat. Slice the strawberries and gently mix into the salad with the oil and juice. Serve on a bed of rocket.

29. Chicken Skewers with Satay Sauce

Ingredients:

5 oz pigeon breast, dig chunks 1 tsp. Ground turmeric 1/2 tsp. extra virgin vegetable oil

1.5 oz Buckwheat

1 oz Kale, stalks removed and sliced 1 oz Celery, sliced

4 Walnut halves, chopped, to garnish

¼ purple onion , diced 1 clove , chopped

1 tsp. Extra virgin vegetable oil 1 tsp. favorer

1 tsp. Ground turmeric

¼ cup chicken broth ½ cup Coconut milk

1 tbsp. Walnut butter or spread 1 tbsp. Coriander, chopped

Directions:

Mix the chicken with the turmeric and vegetable oil and put aside to marinate 30 minutes to 1 hour would be best, but if you're short on time, just leave it for as long as you'll

Cook the buckwheat consistent with the packet instruc tions, for the last 5-7 minutes of cooking time, the kale and celery are added. Drain. Heat the grill on a high setting.

For the sauce, gently fry the purple onion and garlic within the vegetable oil for 2–3 minutes until soft. Add the spices and cook for an extra minute. Add the stock and coconut milk and convey to the boil, then add the walnut butter and stir through. Reduce the warmth and simmer the sauce for 8 or 10 minutes, or till creamy and rich. As the sauce is simmering, thread the chicken on to the skewers and place under the recent grill for 10 minutes, turning them after 5 minutes. To serve, stir the coriander through the sauce and pour it over the skewers, then scatter over the chopped walnuts.

30. Smoked salmon omelette

Ingredients:

2 Medium eggs

4 oz Smoked salmon, sliced 1/2 tsp. Capers

0.5 oz Rocket, chopped 1 tsp. Parsley, chopped

1 tsp. Extra virgin olive oil

Directions:

Crack the eggs into a bowl and whisk well. Add the salmon, capers, rocket and parsley.

Heat the olive oil during a non-stick frypan until hot but not smoking. Add the egg mixture and, employing a spatula or turner, move the mixture round the pan until it's even. Reduce the warmth and let the omelette cook through. Slide the spatula around the edges and roll up or fold the omelette in half to serve.

31. The Sirtfood Diet's Shakshuka

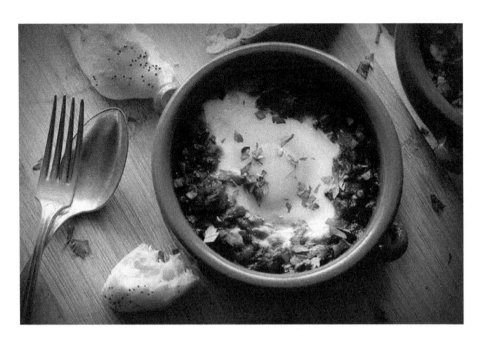

Ingredients:

1 tsp. extra virgin vegetable oil

½ purple onion, finely chopped 1 Garlic clove, finely chopped 1 oz Celery, finely chopped

1 Bird's eye chilli, finely chopped 1 tsp. Groud cumin 1 tsp. Ground turmeric 1 tsp. Paprika

3 Tinned chopped tomatoes

1 oz Kale, stems removed and roughly chopped 1 tbsp. Chopped parsley 2 Medium eggs D

Directions:

Heat alittle , deep-sided frypan over a medium–low heat. Add the oil and fry the onion, garlic, celery, chilli and spices for 1–2 minutes.

Add the tomatoes, then leave the sauce to simmer gently for 20 minutes, stirring occasionally.

Add the kale and cook for an extra 5 minutes. If you are feeling the sauce is getting too thick, simply add a touch water. When your sauce features a nice rich consistency, stir within the parsley.

Make two little wells within the sauce and crack each egg into them. Reduce the heat to its lowest setting and canopy the pan with a lid or foil. Leave the eggs to cook for 10–12 minutes, at which point the whites should be firm while the yolks are still runny. Cook for a further 3–4 minutes if you favor the yolks to be firm. Serve immediately – ideally straight from the pan.

32. Chicken with Broccoli & Mushrooms

Preparation time: **15 minutes**

Cooking time: **25 minutes**

Servings: 6

Ingredients

3 tablespoons olive oil

1 pound skinless, boneless chicken breast, cubed

1 medium onion, chopped

6 garlic cloves, minced

2 cups fresh mushrooms, sliced

16 ounces small broccoli florets

¼ cup water

Salt and ground black pepper, to taste

Directions

1. Over medium heat, heat the oil in a large wok and cook the chicken cubes for around 4-5 minutes.

2. With a slotted spoon, transfer the chicken cubes onto a plate.

3. In the same wok, add the onion and sauté for about 4–5 minutes.

4. Add the fungus and cook for approximately 4-5 minutes.

5. Stir in the cooked chicken, broccoli, and water, and cook (covered) for about 8–10 minutes, stirring occasionally.

6. Stir in salt and black pepper and remove from heat.

7. Serve hot.

33. Buckwheat noodles with chicken kale & miso dressing

Ingredients

For the noodles:

2-3 handfuls of kale leaves

5 oz buckwheat noodles (100% buckwheat, no wheat) 3-4 shiitake mushrooms, sliced

1 tsp copra oil or ghee

1 brown onion, finely diced

1 medium free-range pigeon breast , sliced or diced 1 long red chilli, thinly sliced

2 large garlic cloves, finely diced2-3 tbsp Tamari sauce (gluten-free soy sauce)

For the miso

dressing: 1½ tablespoon fresh organic miso 1 tbsp Tamari sauce

1 tbsp extra-virgin vegetable oil 1 tbsp lemon or juice

1 tsp sesame oil (optional)

Directions:

Bring an medium saucepan of water to boil. Add the kale and cook for 1 minute, until slightly wilted. Remove and set aside but reserve the water and convey it back to the boil. Add the soba noodles and cook consistent with the package instructions (usually about 5 minutes). Rinse under cold water and put aside.

Within the meantime, pan fry the shiitake mushrooms during a little ghee or coconut oil (about a teaspoon) for 2-3 minutes, until lightly browned on all sides. Sprinkle with sea salt and put aside.

Within the same frypan , heat more copra oil or ghee over medium-high heat. Sauté onion and chilli for 2-3 minutes and then add the chicken pieces. Cook 5 minutes over medium heat, stirring a couple of times, then add the garlic, tamari sauce and a touch splash of water. Cook for a further 2-3 minutes, stirring frequently until chicken is cooked through.

Finally, add the kale and soba noodles and toss through the chicken to warm up.
Mix the miso dressing and drizzle over the noodles right at the end of cooking, this manner you'll keep all those beneficial probiotics in the miso alive and active.

34. Baked salmon salad (creamy mint dressing)

Ingredients:

1 salmon fillet (4 oz)

1.5 oz mixed salad leaves

1.5 oz young spinach leaves

2 radishes, trimmed and thinly sliced 2 oz cucumber, dig chunks

2 spring onions, trimmed and sliced

1 small handful parsley, roughly chopped

For the dressing:

1 tsp low-fat mayonnaise 1 tbsp natural yogurt

1 tbsp rice vinegar

2 leaves mint, finely chopped

Salt and freshly ground black pepper

Directions:

Preheat the oven to 390 °F.

Place the salmon fillet on a baking tray and bake for 16–18 minutes until just cooked through. Remove from the oven and set aside. The salmon is equally nice hot or cold in the salad. If your salmon has skin, simply cook skin side down and remove the salmon from the skin employing a turner after cooking. It should slide off easily when cooked.

During a small bowl, mix together the mayonnaise, yogurt, rice wine vinegar, mint leaves and salt and pepper together and leave to face for a minimum of 5 minutes to permit the flavors to develop.

Arrange the salad leaves and spinach on a serving plate and top with the radishes, cucumber, spring onions and parsley. Flake the cooked salmon onto the salad and drizzle the dressing over.

35. Choco chip granola

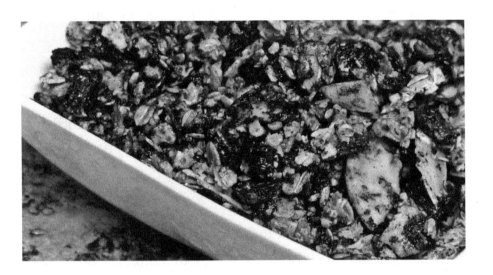

Ingredients:

7 oz jumbo oats

2 oz pecans, roughly chopped 3 tbsp light vegetable oil

1 oz butter

1 tbsp dark sugar

2 tbsp rice malt syrup

2 oz good-quality (70%) bittersweet chocolate chips

Direction:

Preheat the oven to 320 °F. Line an outsized baking tray with a silicone sheet or baking parchment.

Mix the oats and pecans together during a large bowl. During a small nonstick pan, gently heat the olive oil, butter, sugar and rice malt syrup until the butter has melted and therefore the sugar and syrup have dissolved. Don't allow to boil. Pour the syrup over the oats and stir thoroughly until the oats are fully covered.

Distribute the granola over the baking tray, spreading right into the corners. Leave clumps of mixture with spacing instead of an even spread. Bake within the oven for 20 minutes until just tinged golden brown at the edges. Remove from the oven and leave to chill on the tray completely.

When cool, hack any bigger lumps on the tray together with your fingers and then mix within the chocolate chips. Scoop or pour the granola into an airtight tub or jar. The granola will keep for a minimum of 2 weeks.

36. Chargrilled beef

Ingredients:

1 potato, peeled, and dig small dice 1 tbsp extra virgin olive oil

1 tbsp parsley, finely chopped

½ red onion, sliced into rings 2 oz kale, sliced

1 clove, finely chopped

4 oz 1½"-thick beef fillet steak or 1"-thick beefsteak 3 tbsp red wine

½ cup beef broth 1 tsp tomato purée

1 tsp cornflour, dissolved in 1 tbsp water

Directions:

Heat the oven to 430 °F.

Place the potatoes during a saucepan of boiling water, bring back to the boil and cook for 4–5 minutes, then drain. Place during a roasting tin with 1 teaspoon of the oil and roast in the hot oven for 35–45 minutes. Turn the potatoes every 10 minutes to make sure even cooking. When cooked, remove from the oven, sprinkle with the chopped parsley and mix well.

Fry the onion in 1 teaspoon of the oil over medium heat for 5–7 minutes, until soft and nicely caramelized. Keep warm. Steam the kale for 2–3 minutes then drain. Fry the garlic gently in ½ teaspoon of oil for 1 minute, till soft but not colored. Add the kale and fry for a further 1–2 minutes, until tender. Keep warm.

Heat an ovenproof frypan over high heat until smoking. Coat the meat in ½ a teaspoon of the oil and fry within the hot pan over an medium–high heat consistent with how you wish your meat done.If you like your meat medium, it might be better to sear the meat then transfer the pan to an oven set at 430°F and finish the cooking that the way for the prescribed times.

Remove the meat from the pan and set aside to rest. Add the wine to the hot pan to mention any meat residue — Bubble to scale back the wine by half, until syrupy and with a concentrated flavor. Add the stock and tomato purée to the steak pan and convey to the boil, then add the cornflour paste to thicken your sauce, adding it a little at a time until you've got your desired consistency. Stir in any of the juices from the rested steak and serve with the roasted potatoes, kale, onion rings and wine sauce.

37. Greek Sea Bass Mix

Preparation time: 10 minutes

Cooking time: 22 minutes

Servings: 2

Ingredients:

2 sea bass fillets, boneless

1 garlic clove, minced

5 cherry tomatoes, halved

1 tablespoon chopped parsley

2 shallots, chopped

Juice of ½ lemon

1 tablespoon olive oil

8 ounces baby spinach

Cooking spray

Directions:

1. Grease a baking dish with cooking oil then add the fish, tomatoes, parsley and garlic. Drizzle the lemon juice over the fish, cover the dish and place it in the oven at 350 degrees F. Bake for 15 minutes and then divide between plates. Heat a pan over medium heat with the olive oil, add shallot, stir and cook for 1 minute. Add spinach, stir, cook for 5 minutes more, add to the plate with the fish and serve.

38. Veal Cabbage Rolls – Smarter with Capers, Garlic and Caraway Seeds

Ingredients:

1 kg white cabbage (1 white cabbage)

Salt

2 onions

1 clove of garlic

3 tbsp oil

700 g veal mince (request from the butcher)

40 g escapades (glass; depleted weight)

2 eggs Pepper

1 tsp favorer

1 tbsp paprika powder (sweet)

400 ml veal stock

125 ml soy cream

Directions:

Wash the cabbage and evacuate the external leaves. Cut out the tail during a wedge. Spot a huge pot of salted water and heat it to the aim of boiling. Within the interim, expel 16 leaves from the cabbage during a gentle progression, increase the bubbling water and cook for 3-4 minutes

Lift out, flush under running virus water and channel. Spot on a kitchen towel, spread with a subsequent towel and pat dry Cut out the hard, center leaf ribs.

Peel and finely cleave onions and garlic. Warmth 1 tablespoon of oil. Braise the onions and garlic until translucent.

Let cool during a bowl. Include minced meat, tricks, eggs, salt, and pepper and blend everything into a meat player.

Put 2 cabbage leaves together and put 1 serving of mince on each leaf. Move up firmly and fasten it with kitchen string.

Heat the rest of the oil during a pan and earthy colored the 8 cabbage abounds in it from all sides.

Add the caraway and paprika powder. Empty veal stock into the pot and heat to the aim of boiling. Cover and braise the cabbage turns over medium warmth for 35–40 minutes, turn within the center. Mix the soy cream into the sauce and let it bubble for an extra 5 minutes. Season with salt and pepper. Put the cabbage roulades on a plate and present with earthy colored rice or pureed potatoes.

39. Prawns Sweet and Spicy Glaze with China-Cole-Slav

Ingredients:

250 g Chinese cabbage (0.25 Chinese cabbage)

Salt

50 g little carrots (1 little carrot)

1 little red onion

½ lime

75 ml coconut milk (9% fat)

2 tsp sugar

1 tsp vinegar

Pepper

2 stems coriander

3 tbsp pure sweetener

1 dried stew pepper

2 tbsp Thai fish sauce

1 clove of garlic

3 spring onions

400 g shrimps (with shell, 8 shrimps)

2 tbsp oil

Directions:

Clean the cabbage and evacuate the tail. Cut the cabbage into fine strips over the rib. Sprinkle with somewhat salt, blend vivaciously and let steep for half-hour.

Within the interim, strip the carrot, dig fine strips. Strip the red onion and furthermore dig strips. Crush the lime.

Mix coconut milk with sugar, vinegar, 1 tbsp juice, and slightly pepper. Channel the cabbage and blend it in with the carrot and onion strips with the coconut milk.

Wash the coriander leaves, shake dry, pluck the leaves, cleave and blend within the plate of mixed greens. Let it steep for an extra half-hour.

Boil the natural sweetener, stew pepper, fish sauce, and three tablespoons of water during a touch pot and cook while mixing until the sugar has totally weakened. Allow chill to off.

Peel and smash garlic. The spring onions are washed and cleaned and cut into pieces about 2 cm long.

Break the shrimp out of the shells, however, leave the rear ends on the shrimp.

Cut open the rear, evacuate the dark digestion tracts. Wash shrimp and pat dry.

Heat oil within the wok and to the aim of smoke. Include the shrimp and garlic and fry quickly. Season with pepper.

Add 3-4 tablespoons of the bean stew fish sauce and cook while mixing until the sauce adheres to the shrimp; that takes around 2 minutes.

Add the onion pieces and fry for an extra 45 seconds. Season the coleslaw once more. Put the shrimp on a plate and present it with the serving of mixed greens.

40. Vegetarian Lasagna - Smarter with Seitan and Spinach

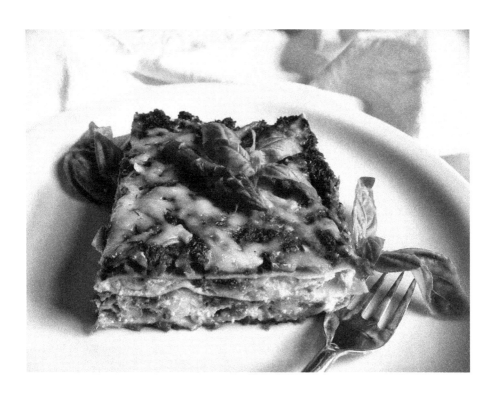

Ingredients:

225 g spinach leaves (solidified)

300 g seitan

2nd little carrots

2 sticks celery

1 onion

1 clove of garlic

2 tbsp oil Salt Pepper

850 g canned tomatoes

200 ml exemplary vegetable stock

1 tsp fennel seeds

30 g parmesan (1 piece)

Nutmeg

225 g ricotta

16 entire grain lasagna sheets

Butter for the form

150 g mozzarella

Directions:

Let the spinach defrost. Hack the seitan finely or put it through the center cut of the meat processor.

Wash and strip carrots. Wash, clean, expel, and finely dice the celery. Strip and cleave the onion and garlic.

Heat the oil during a pan and braise the carrots, celery, onions, and garlic for 3 minutes over medium warmth. Include from that point forward and braise for 3 minutes while mixing. Season with salt and pepper.

Put the canned tomatoes and stock within the pan and spread and cook over medium warmth for 20 minutes, mixing every so often. Pulverize the fennel seeds, include, and season the sauce with salt and pepper.

Meanwhile, finely grind the Parmesan. Concentrate on some nutmeg. Crush the spinach enthusiastically, generally slash, and blend during a bowl with the ricotta, parmesan, salt, pepper, and nutmeg.

Lightly oil a preparing dish (approx. 30 x 20 cm). Spread rock bottom of the shape with slightly sauce and smooth it out. Spot 4 sheets of lasagna on the brink of every other, if essential slice to estimate. Add 1/3 of the spinach blend and smooth. Spread 1/4 of the sauce on top. Layer 4 lasagna sheets, 1/3 spinach, and 1/4 sauce once more, rehash the procedure. Place the keep going lasagna sheets on top and spread the remainder of the sauce over them.

Drain the mozzarella and attack enormous pieces. Spread on the lasagna. Heat veggie-lover lasagna during a preheated stove at 180 ° C (fan broiler: 160 ° C, gas: levels 2–3) on the center rack for 35–40 minutes. Let the veggie lover lasagna rest for around 5 minutes before serving.

41. Asparagus and Ham Omelet with Potatoes and Parsley

Ingredients:

200 g new potatoes

Salt

150 g white asparagus

1 onion

50 g bresaola (Italian meat ham)

2 stems parsley

3 eggs

1 tbsp rapeseed oil

Pepper

Directions:

Wash the potatoes well. Cook in bubbling salted water for approx. 20 minutes, channel and let cool. While the potatoes are cooking, strip the asparagus, remove the lower woody closures. Cook asparagus in salted water for around quarter-hour, scoop of the water, channel well and let cool. Strip the onion and hack finely.

Cut the asparagus and potatoes into little pieces.

Cut the bresaola into strips.

Wash parsley, shake dry, pluck leaves, and slash. Beat the eggs during a bowl and race with the hacked parsley.

Heat the oil during a covered skillet and sauté the onion solid shapes until medium-high warmth until translucent.

Add potatoes and keep it up simmering for 2 minutes.

Add asparagus and fry for 1 moment.

Add the bresaola and season everything with salt and pepper.

Put the eggs within the skillet and spread and stew for 5–6 minutes over low warmth. Drop out of the skillet and serve directly.

42. Poached Eggs on Spinach with sauce

Ingredients:

1 clove of garlic

3 tsp. oil

1 tsp. sugar

200 ml wine

Salt

Pepper

1 shallot

250 g youthful spinach leaves

Nutmeg

2 tbsp vinegar

4 eggs

2 cuts entire grain toast

Directions:

Peel and finely slash the garlic and braise in 1 teaspoon of oil. Sprinkle sugar, include wine, and convey to the bubble. Lessen to 1/3 over medium warmth. Salt, pepper and keep warm.

Peel the shallot and shakers finely. Wash the spinach well and let it channel. Warmth the rest of the oil during a skillet, sauté the shallot during a smooth warmth. Include the spinach and let it a breakdown in 3-4 minutes. Include slightly nutmeg, salt, and pepper.

Boil 1 liter of water with the vinegar. Painstakingly beat the eggs during a bowl with the goal that the yolks stay flawless.

Stir the bubbling vinegar water energetically with a whisk.

Now let the eggs slide in (by the pivot of the water they separate right away). Boil the water once more. Expel the pot from the hob at that point and allow the eggs to cook for 3-4 minutes (poach).

Scoop the eggs with a froth trowel and permit them to channel. Put the spinach on a plate and put the eggs thereon. Shower with the sauce and serve. Toast the bread within the toaster and present with it.

43. Pasta with Minced Lamb Balls and Eggplant, Tomatoes and Sultanas

Ingredients:

250 gleans minced sheep

2 tbsp low-fat quark

1 egg

2 tbsp breadcrumbs

Salt

Pepper

1 tsp. cinnamon

200 g little eggplant (1 little eggplant)

1 onion

1 clove of garlic

2 tbsp oil

150 g orecchiette pasta

2 tbsp sultanas

400 g pizza tomatoes (can)

1 straight leaf

125 ml great vegetable stock

Directions:

Mix minced sheep, quark, egg, and breadcrumbs during a bowl. Season with salt, pepper, and cinnamon.

Using wet hands, transform the slash into balls the size of a cherry. Chill quickly.

Clean, wash, dry the eggplant, and dig 5 mm blocks. Strip onion and garlic and hack finely.

Heat 1 tablespoon of oil during a skillet and fry the meatballs in it until brilliant earthy colored. Expel and put during a secure spot.

Wipe out the dish and afterward heat up the rest of the oil. Include the eggplant shapes, onion, and garlic and braise for 4-5 minutes, mixing. Meanwhile, cook the pasta nibble verification during tons of bubbling salted water as per the bundle guidelines.

Add the sultanas, tomatoes, and sound leave to the skillet. Pour within the stock and convey it to the bubble.

Cover and cook for 4 minutes over medium warmth. At that point put the meatballs within the dish and cook secured for an extra 5

44. Vegetable Spaghetti

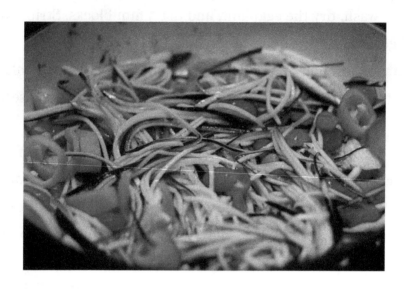

Ingredients:

200 g red chime pepper (1 red ringer pepper)

200 g yellow chime pepper (1 yellow ringer pepper)

150 g carrots (2 carrots)

300 g broccoli

12 yellow cherry tomatoes

½ pack parsley

20 g tawny (8 leaves)

3 spring onions

300 g entire grain spaghetti

Salt

½ lemon

4 tbsp oil Pepper

Directions:

Quarter the peppers, center them, wash and spot them on a heating sheet, skin side up. Broil under the recent flame broil until the skin turns dark and rankles.

Cover and let cool during a bowl secured for 10 minutes (steam). At that point skin and dig fine strips.

Peel the carrots and cut them into flimsy cuts.

Clean broccoli, dig little florets and wash. Wash and split tomatoes.

Clean the parsley, shake it out, pick up the leaves, clean and wash roan, generally hack both. The spring onions are cleaned, washed and cut into meager cuts.

Cook the spaghetti nibble evidence during tons of salted water as indicated by the bundle directions. Include broccoli and carrots 4 minutes before the finish of the cooking time.

Squeeze lemon. Channel the pasta and blend during a bowl with the readied Ingredients:, 1 teaspoon lemon squeeze, and oil.

45. Spaghetti with Salmon in Lemon Sauce

Ingredients:

150 g salmon filet (without skin)

100 g leek (1 flimsy stick)

100 g little carrots (2 little carrots)

½ natural lemon

2 stems parsley

150 g entire grain spaghetti Salt

2 tbsp oil Pepper

100 ml of fish stock

150 ml of soy cream

Directions:

Wash salmon, pat dry, and dig 2 cm 3D squares.

The leek is dried, washed and cut into dainty circles. Strip the carrots and cut them into flimsy strips.

Within the interim, wash the lemon half hot and rub dry. Strip the lemon strip meagerly and dig fine strips. Crush juice. Wash parsley, shake dry, pluck leaves and cleave finely.

Cook the pasta chomp verification in saltwater as indicated by the bundle guidelines.

Heat oil during a dish. Season the salmon with pepper and fry everywhere within the recent oil for 3-4 minutes.

Remove the salmon, braise the leek rings, and carrot strips within the dish over medium warmth for 3-4 minutes.

Remove the salmon, braise the leek rings, and carrot strips within the dish over medium warmth for 3-4 minutes.

If fundamental, salt the salmon, set it back within the container, and warmth quickly. Blend within the parsley. Drain the pasta during a strainer and blend tenderly with the sauce. Season with salt and pepper and directly serve the spaghetti and salmon.

46. Kale and red onion dahl with Buckwheat

Ingredients::
one tablespoon olive oil
One very little very little onion sliced
Two cm ginger grated
One eye chilli deseeded and finely cleaved (more on the off likelihood that you just that you just things hot!)
two teaspoons turmeric
Two teaspoons garam masala
One hundred sixty g very little lentils
four hundred cc cc milk
two hundred cc cc
A hundred g kale or spinach would be a unprecedented unprecedented One hundred sixty g buckwheat or brown rice

Directions:
Place the olive oil in a very vast, deep saucepan and embody the cut onion.

Cook on a low heat, with the lid on for 5.
Add the garlic, ginger and chilli and cook for one more minute.
Add the turmeric, garam masala and a splash of water and cook for one a lot of a lot of.
Add the red lentils, coconut milk, and 200ml water (do this simply by half filling embody coconut milk can with water and

tipping it into the saucepan). Combine everything together altogether and embody for twenty 5 associate degree a twenty heat with the cover cover. Stir once throughout a jiffy and embody water if the dhal starts to stick.

After twenty minutes add the kale, stir thoroughly and replace the cover, embody for a further five 5 7. About fifteen ready, place embody buckwheat in a medium pot and add plenty of effervescent water. Bring the water back dahl the boil and cook for ten minutes

47. Buckwheat food Salad-Sirt Food Recipes

Ingridients:

50g buckwheat pasta (cooked according to the packet guidelines) Large handful of rocket

Small bunch of basil leaves

Eight cherry tomatoes, halved

1/2 avocado, diced

Ten olives

one tbsp extra virgin edible fat

20g pine loco

Directions:

Gently combine all the ingredients except the pine nuts and arrange on a plate or in a bowl, then scatter the pine nuts over the top.

48. Greek dish Skewers

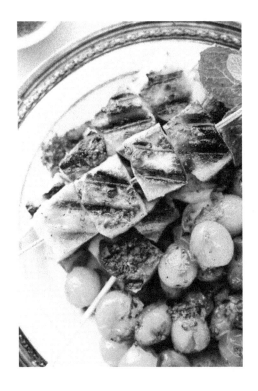

306 Calories,

3.5 of your SIRT five a day,

Serves 2

Ready place 10 5

Ingredients:

Two wood wood, soaked in water cookery 30 minutes before use

Eight vast dark olives

Eight cherry tomatoes

One yellow pepper, cut into eight squares

½ red onion hamper the middle the middle into eight items

100g (about 10cm) cucumber, dig four cuts and halved 100g feta, cut into eight cubes

For the dressing:

one tbsp to boot further olive oil associate degree of ½ half One tsp oleoresin vinegar

½ clove garlic, peeled and press

Few leaves basil, finely chopped (or ½ tsp dried mingling to replace basil and oregano)

Few leaves oregano, finely hacked

Generous seasoning of salt and freshly ground dark pepper

Directions:

Thread each skewer with the salad Ingredients: place the order: olive, tomato, yellow pepper, red onion, cucumber, feta, tomato, olive, yellow pepper, red onion, cucumber, and feta.

Place all the dressing Ingredients: place a small bowl and mix together thoroughly. Pour associate degree the sticks.

49. Kale, Edamame and curd Curry-Sirt Food Recipes

Ingredients:
One tbsp oilseed oil
One large onion, hacked
Four garlic, stripped and three
One vast thumb (7cm) new ginger, peeled and ground One red
stew, deseeded and thinly sliced 1/2 tsp ground turmeric
1/4 tsp cayenne pepper
One tsp paprika
1/2 one ground cumin
one tsp salt
250g dried two lentils
One litre boiling water
50g frozen soyaedamame beans
200g firm tofu, hacked into cubes
Two tomatoes, roughly hacked
Juice of one embody
200g kale leaves, stalks expelled and torn

Directions
Place the oil place associate degree associate degree associate
degree associate degree a low-medium heat. Embody the
embody and embody for 5 5 5 5 the three, ginger and stew and

preparation preparation a preparation two preparation. Embody the turmeric, cayenne, paprika, cumin and salt. Stir through 5 5 the red lentils and stirring once more.

Pour in the boiling water and bring Cajanus cajan a hearty simmer for ten minutes, then reduce the heat and cook for a further 20-30 minutes till the curry options an options options consistency.

Add the soya beans, bean curd and tomatoes and cook preparation a preparation five preparation. Embody embody embody juice and kale leaves and cook till embody kale is just tender.

50. Sirt Food Miso Marinated Cod with herb

Serves 1

Ingredients:

20g miso

One tbsp mirin

One tbsp extra virgin olive oil

200g skinless cod filet

20g two onion, sliced

40g celery, sliced

One garlic clove, finely chopped

One bird's eye bean stew, finely chopped One one finely slashed

new ginger 60g inexperienced beans

50g kale, typically chopped

One tsp herb herb

5g parsley, typically chopped

one tbsp tamari

30g buckwheat

one tsp ground turmeric

Directions:

Mix the miso, mirin and one teaspoon two the oil. Rub all over the cod and leave to marinate for thirty thirty. Heat the oven Cajanus cajan 220°C/gas seven.

Bake the cod preparation ten preparation.

Meanwhile, heat an associate degree cooking pan or cooking pan with embody cooking pan oil. Embody the onion and pan deep-fried food for a number of of moments, then add the celery, garlic, chilli, ginger, green beans and kale. Toss and fry 5 the kale is tender and grilled grilled. You may need to include slightly to help to help process.

Cook the buckwheat according to the bundle instructions with the turmeric for three 5.

Add the sesame seeds, parsley and tamari to embody pan sear and serve with embody greens and fish.